# PALEO DIET:

A Quick and Easy Guide for Beginners: The Secrets of
Rapid Weight Loss and a Healthy Lifestyle.

Sarah Maddington

Table of Contents

# About Sarah Maddington

Sarah Maddington was born and raised in Manchester, UK. She is a Weight-Loss coach, Dietitian, Professional Chef and a mother of two. After finishing high school, she moved to London to pursue her dreams to study culinary.

In the past, Sarah was very overweight and suffered many health problems. She struggled with weight issues and found it difficult to maintain the balance between her career and her health.

It wasn't until after giving birth to her eldest daughter Sally, did she realise that she had to take her health more seriously if she wanted to become a role model for her children.
She lost 57 pounds in 6 months. Today, she wants to inspire beautiful people around the world to take control of the health so they can get back the life they deserve.

# Introduction

It's easy to raise an eyebrow when you hear the term paleo diet. Many people assume it's just another diet with a poorly thought out weight loss scheme, but it's not some gimmick or fad that will fade away. It's just a return to the diet that nature intended for us to have. It traces back to the days of our ancestors where we were hunter and gatherers during a paleolithic Era. A paleo diet consists of dietary stables such as seeds, nuts, berries, and fresh meat.

A paleo diet, much like the Atkins diet, will cut out most of your carbs. However, unlike the Atkins diet which will focus on how many carbs you cut from your day to day meals, a paleo diet will focus more on your overall health. The Atkins diet encourages people to gorge on meats even if they have antibiotics or hormones used. A paleo diet requires that you eat healthy meats that are hormone free and grass fed.

There are studies that suggest it is not a coincidence that Atkin dieters suffer from heart attacks. This diet even allows you to gorge on fatty meats such as bacon, which is soaked in grease and sure to leave you with clogged arteries despite how thin someone may be. In short, the Atkins diet can increase your cholesterol and contribute to heart disease.

However, paleo diets do not have the same pit falls since it concentrates on more than just the reduction of carbs. It also concentrates on the actual nutrients that you're putting into your body. It doesn't matter how many low carb and low fat foods you eat if the nutrient value isn't what you need for your body. You'll still be unhealthy. Like every organism on the planet, our bodies and the needs our bodies have, has been defined and developed over time, and it is important that we address those needs properly.

Naturally, food is available that has the nutrients we need, but we've come to depend on foods that are not organic, fed improperly, grown through modification, or even injected with hormones. Our paleo ancestors lived 150,000 years before the modern conveniences and interference with our food, and they had no issue getting the nutrients they needed to not just survive, but thrive with healthy, abled bodies. With proper care, you can get these nutrients too, and build a happier, healthier you.

# Chapter 1: What is a Paleo Diet?

Dr. Walter Voegtlin endorses a paleolithic lifestyle as a dietary concept in his book, *The Stone Age Diet,* which was release in 1975. This book paved way for what are now considered Paleolothic advances, which are similar to the core beliefs of our ancestors with variosu limitations and regulations.

To understand paleo diets, you must first understand a paleolithic period, which was pre-agriculture during the majority of it's time. There are many foods that we eat in large quantities that our Paleolithic ancestors would eat in their unprocessed form. Therefore, our ancestors gained more nutrients from these foods. When we go back to consuming these foods in the same way as our ancestors, then you are partaking in a paleo diet. You need to be selective when pricking up authentic, unprocessed food also known as whole foods.

By eating whole foods you eliminate additives, sugars and salts that are included in processed foods, which can actually be highly addicting. By going from processed foods to actual whole food, you're going to feel healthier and make healthier eating habits. It is best that a paleo dieter tries to eat as organically as they can. Choose grass fed meats over farm raised, select various fruits and vegetables, and try to stick with natural foods such as nuts and seeds. Of course, there are more lenient adaptations which will allow you to eat certain prohibited foods such as yams, low-fat dairy goods, and fruits and vegetables that have a high level of fructose. These foods were not originally accessible during the Palelothic era.

Supporters of paleo diets believe that our digestive system has not evolved significantly since a paleolthic era, so certain foods cause gastrointestinal pain and pressure.

These foods include:

- Legumes
- Cereal & Grains

- Starchy Vegetables
- All Processed Foods
- Table Salt
- All Dairy
- Processed Sugar
- Distilled vegetable oils

There are different versions of paleo diets that offer different limits, so find the one that's best for you. This is why some versions allow for low-fat dairy products, yams, and other foods. However, all versions of paleo diets promote you eating vegetables, fruits, and lean proteins. It's important that you get your good fat from natural sources such as nuts, with the exception of peanuts, grass-fed meat and seeds.

Due to the strict limitations of what you can and can't eat, a paleo diet is low on carbs but full of healthy fats and proteins, which will provide your body with the necessary vitamins, minerals, fiber and phytochemicals it needs to function. Though, keep in mind you cannot have seasoned cold cut meats, but you can have fruits and vegetables that have alkaline, which is different than various traditional diets. Fat is necessary to the human body, so a paleo diet does not exclude it. Instead, it provides you with natural fats that come from seafood, fish, grass-fed cattle, nuts, seeds, and other natural oils that aid in our digestive system. Due to the lack of grains, dairy, processed food, and sugar, a paleo diet often leads to weight loss too.

# Chapter 2: Going a paleo Way

A paleo diet requires that you avoid potatoes, grains, and legumes, dairy, and refined or processed products. You'll also need to avoid most vegetable oils and any refined sugars. Instead, you'll introduce fruits, vegetables, fish, and grass-fed meats to your table. You'll need to procure organic produce, and it's even better if you can get it locally sourced! It's a common misconception that a paleo diet requires you to stick to a raw-food diet. Your food can be eaten raw or cooked, and it's important that you keep a variety in your meal plans. This will keep you from becoming bored with your diet, and it'll allow you to maintain the proper balance of vitamins and minerals that your body needs to stay healthy.

## Some Health Benefits

There are many benefits to a paleo diet, and you'll find most of them listed below.

- **Weight Loss & Toning:** A paleo diet will reduce the amount of stored fat on your body because of how you'll be eating, which will help you to shed those pounds and tone up.
- **Antioxidants & Vitamins:** The food you'll be eating is full of phytonutrients, antioxidants and other vitamins that you need. A large amount of your vitamins will come from the necessary fruit you'll be introducing to your day to day meals.
- **Improved Brain Function:** Since a paleo diet provides essential proteins and vitamins, including omega-3s due to the high fish content, your brain will be getting the critical fatty acids it needs for development. It can also lead to a healthy heart and eyes!

The best part is that you don't need to count your calories with a paleo diet! Instead, you're just controlling your portions. Prehistoric men never counted their calories and they didn't need to when they were eating healthy and eating to survive. Instead, you'll rely on the nutrients in your food to keep you from gaining weight and to provide you with their numerous health benefits.

Clean out the pantry because all processed foods have to go! Yes, all of it. Say goodbye to the potato chips, Little Debbie's, and more. You have to clean your body out, and make sure that it gets rid of all the additional fuel that it's stored in in the way of fat. You'll find that various modern diseases can be prevented just by eating healthy, so there's no reason to complicate your life with food that's bad for you.  It's all about natural food, to return your body to natural working order.

# Paleo Diet FAQs

In this chapter, you'll learn the answer too many frequently asked questions about a paleo diet, so let's dive right in!

## Is this diet a scam?

 The simple answer is no it isn't. Humans only at what they could forage or hunt for 140,000 years. This means that their diet consisted of vegetables, nuts, fruits, meat and fish. Grains weren't even thought of as a food source, and therefore there is a reason that grains are cut out of a paleo diet. This type of diet worked for our ancestors, and it's considered a natural way to eat. The human body was designed for this type of diet, which is why it works! A paleo diet is all about getting your body back on the diet it was designed for from the start.

## Will it actually work?

There are studies that support that paleo diets actually work because it's full of clean, healthy and unprocessed food. When you cut out carbs and sugars, you're going to lessen your bloating and lose weight. You'll feel and be healthier this way! You're also cutting out the chemicals that come with processed foods. You're loading up on healthy fats and proteins, so that you feel fuller for longer and actually eat less too. You'll even have a wider options of healthy fibers due to the large amount of fruits and vegetables that the diet calls for. You'll even get all of the vitamins and minerals you need right from your food, which will boost your energy levels. So say goodbye to energy drinks and the need for caffeine, because a paleo diet will provide you with everything that you need.

## How much weight can you lose with this diet?

This all depends on the person because each person reacts to diets differently. Not everyone has gained weight for the same reason either. The reason you gained weight will determine how you lose it. For example, if most of your weight comes from water retention, cutting down the salt which help. If most of it comes from processed foods, a paleo diet is sure to help. If it comes from a sugar addiction, then you'll lose more by cutting out the sugary culprits. You can lose anything from five to ten pounds in the first week, but keep in mind that some of it may be water weight. After the first week, it's common for your weight loss to be taper off to one to three pounds a week. Your body will naturally shed the weight on this diet, but how much depends on the person. Your fat cells will start to shrink, and you won't even need to cut back your calories! Slow and steady isn't just the way to win the race, but it's actually healthier for you in the long run.


## How long do I have to wait for results?

Most people start to see weight loss results within the first week of starting their new paleo diet. Though, some people will lose more than others. After the first two weeks, you can expect those results to slow down, but they will not stop altogether.


## What foods am I allowed?

You're encouraged to eat fish, seafood, grass-fed meat, fresh vegetables, eggs, seeds and nuts, fresh fruits, sweet potatoes, yams, and healthy oils on a paleo diet. Healthy oils include olive oil, walnut oil, flaxseed oil, avocado oil, macadamia oil, and coconut oil. Many people will subsite coconut or almond milk for their dairy as well, which will make your dairy paleo approved, which is good news for any dairy lover that still wants to benefit from a paleo lifestyle. You can also have natural sweeteners such as pure maple syrup and honey.

## Is this diet safe as well as healthy?

A paleo diet is considered to be safer than the modern American diet because you are not relying on processed foods, fatty meats, and a limited amount of healthy fat, fruit or vegetables. You'll get the vitamins, fiber, nutrients and minerals that you need from whole, unprocessed food, which will allow you to live a healthy life.

# Chapter 3: The Cause of Success

A paleo diet is a success for many because it puts your body in a fat-burning mode instead of a carbohydrate burning one, which most people are in. when your body is burning fat, you're shedding pounds and using the energy that your body would otherwise store as fat. The ideal source of energy for your body is from fats.

Fat burns slower, and it's easier for your body to utilize fat. However, because of the sheer amount of carbs that the average person eats each and every day, many people have their bodies trained to burn the carbs instead of their fat. People end up eating an excess amount of carbs, which the body cannot burn through in a single day, so that's why it's stored as fat. This was great when people were risking starvation on a regular basis, but when the likelihood of starvation is slim to none, it causes excessive weight gain instead.

This is why most western countries are facing an obesity epidemic. A paleo diet uses a straightforward strategy. Eliminate the plain carbs from your diet so that you can burn the fat that you already have stored and provide your body only with the energy it needs. When your carbs are depleted, your body can escape this cycle, teaching it to burn fat instead.

When your body no longer has a steady flow of carbs that it's able to convert to sugar, your blood sugar will slump to a normal point, and then your insulin can work properly to control it. When your insulin is in control, lipolysis can happen. This is the course the body takes when it frees triglycerides, which is used in fat storage, so that your body can burn it as energy. Therefore, cutting down your carb intake will star the fat burning process and lead to noticeable weight loss.

# Chapter 4: What You Can Eat

Figuring out what you can eat is the most important part of going paleo. How else will you know if a recipe or dish can make it to your table?

You can eat almost any nut or seeds, including pecans, pumpkin seeds, walnuts, macadamia nuts, almonds, hazelnuts, cashews, and pine nuts. The only nut you cannot eat is a peanut.

You can eat most meat and fish so long as it is grass-fed. Try to make sure that you aren't getting meat that has been genetically modified or shot up with antibiotics. This includes pork, beef, poultry, buffalo, most fish, lobster, clams, and more.

Remember that you need to keep your beverages paleo friendly too! You'll want to stick with herbal teas, natural fruit juice, vegetable juice, and filtered or natural spring water. Don't drink water where things have been added to it.

What cooking oils you use and the fats you take in are important to. Stick to coconut oil, extra virgin olive oil, avocado oil, walnut oil, hazelnut oil, natural grease, lard and macadamia oil.

While not all vegetables and fruits are paleo friendly, most of them are. Berries of all types are welcome! You can also eat apricots, apple, guava, cantaloupe, papaya, lemon, bananas, mango, oranges, honeydew, peaches, kiwi, tangerines, and melons. You'll also be able to eat watercress, zucchini, tomato, pumpkin, squash, peppers, onions, eggplants, broccoli, celery, beets, asparagus, mustard, carrots, and mushrooms. Greens are a healthy and paleo friendly food too, so make sure to eat Swiss chard, spinach, turnips and turnip greens, and dandelion greens too!

Remember that while processed sugar is not allowed, natural sweeteners are! Try out some raw honey, such as clover honey, wildflower, creamed honey, and orange blossom honey. Pure maple syrup is allowed too!

## Some Basic Guidelines

With every meal you're going to enjoy protein, and you'll need to go overboard with the vegetables and fruit throughout the day. You can eat your vegetables cooked or raw as long as your recipes are paleo friendly! Make sure that you're eating hormone and chemical free, and try to keep your diet low in saturated fat.

You'll want to use sea salt and be reasonable with how much salt you use. Just remember that many condiments are loaded with additives, sodium, and chemicals, so try to use organic seasonings instead. You can make your own condiments and seasoning blends too!

If you exercise, you're going to increase your weight loss too! You'll help your body to produce hormones that will give you the energy you need to get through the day!

Limit your saturated fats as much as possible if you can't cut them out completely! Avocado is usually the best source of healthy fats too! You'll also need to limit how much alcohol you consume. Many people don't care to cut out alcohol completely, but stick to good quality wine and try to keep away from cocktails. Cocktails are laden with artificial ingredients and sugar which certainly goes against a paleo diet.

# Chapter 5: The Foods to Avoid

Knowing what food to avoid can be just as important as knowing which foods are paleo friendly, and that's exactly what this chapter will help you with.

## Avoiding Dairy

Dairy and dairy products may be full of nutrients, but science has proven that the human body has a hard time processing them. Dairy often causes allergic reactions to many, and it can cause severe problems with your digestive system it can also leave people prone to autoimmune diseases. Dairy can also cause inflammation, resulting in skin conditions, headaches and joint pain.

Many people are lactose intolerance as well. To understand lactose intolerance, you need to understand that lactose is a particular type of sugar that resides within milk. It can only be processed if your body is producing the enzyme lactase. Lactose intolerance is due to someone not being able to produce lactase or at least not be able to produce enough of it. The lack of lactase will cause the sugars to ferment in your gut, causing inflammation and discomfort.

Many people are under the misconception that milk is the only source of calcium, but this isn't the case. You do need calcium to develop healthy teeth and bones, but during a paleolithic age dairy wasn't an option. You can get calcium from other foods such as oranges, kale, almonds, spinach and more!

## Why You Need to Eliminate Processed Foods

Processed foods lead to trouble and open you up to a slew of different diseases including hypertension and type-2 diabetes. Even if you don't want to stick to a paleo diet, processed foods have an adverse effect on your overall health. Since processed foods are meant to last on the shelf, they're pumped full of artificial flavors, chemicals and preservatives that your body isn't naturally made to break down. These chemicals, preservatives and artificial flavors will interfere with your weight and your sugar levels. Look at the list on the label. If the list is long, it's likely processed.

## Keep Refined Sugars & Grains Away

All processed sugar is refined sugar, and you need to stay away! In the process of refining, it gets rid of the minerals and nutrients that come with it. Therefore, you can kiss the minerals, vitamins, and protein and fiber content goodbye. You're just getting empty calories that won't assist your body in any ways.

Stay away from artificial sweeteners, brown sugar, high fructose corn syrup, and white table sugar. As well as being full of nothing but empty calories, it also will take minerals and vitamins away from your body because your body has to work to digest it, detox from it, and eliminate it after consumptions. Your energy levels will suffer too! You can use raw honey, coconut syrup and molasses, or pure maple syrup if you're craving something sweet.

# Chapter 6: Some Frugal Shopping Tips

Many people think that a paleo diet is an expensive one, but this doesn't have to
be the case! That's where this chapter comes in handy.

## Tips to Save Money

You can be paleo and frugal too! Just avoid buying excessive amounts of food at
one time, which can be tempting for many people. Some foods will lose their
flavor over time, even if you keep them in your refrigerator. With a paleo diet,
you'll want to shop frequently instead, and try to purchase what's in season if you
want to save some cash!

## Why Buy Seasonally

The prices of groceries vary depending on what season you're in. when something
is out of season, it'll cost more money because it has to be either imported or
grown in a greenhouse. It'll be easier to find times when they're in season too
without having to resort to frozen food. Food that's seasonal is also fresher and
packed full of nutrients and flavor. You may want to start shopping locally too!
Many farmer markets and flea markets that have a local produce section are more
than willing to cut you a deal. If you have the supplies, you may want to freeze
your own fruits and vegetables too, which will save you money in the long run. All
you need is containers and a deep freezer.

## Write it Down

If you don't have a plan, it can be harder to save money when grocery shopping.
Make a list of the items that you need for your meals and schedule in advance. To
do this, try to know what season you're in and what sales your local grocery stores

may be having. Choose versatile vegetables that can go in salads, stir fries, soups and so on so that you have a variety of options. By picking up versatile vegetables, you can cut down on your waste which will cut down on your grocery bill. The same applies to your fruits too! Some fruits can be eaten with meals or on their own, such as apples and pineapples which can be paired with pork. Oranges can make juice, and add flavor to your water, so versatile fruit is important to cut down on your grocery bill!

## Shop Around

Check out your local farmer's market, flea markets and produce stands so that you know the average prices. You should also collect flyers from your local grocery stores to compare prices. Coupons aren't much of an option when you're looking for whole ingredients. When you buy from produce stands, farmer's markets, and flea markets, you'll cut out the middleman which cuts out a lot of the price.

## Grow It Yourself!

If you really want to save money, you might want to consider growing some herbs and vegetables yourself. You can grow fruit too, but it's much more of a commitment. Not only will you save money, but there's satisfaction that comes with eating something that you grew yourself! You may want to start with fresh herbs, tomatoes, lettuce, onions, or even berries, which are considered easy to grow.

## Don't Be Wasteful

Remember that it's important to not be wasteful with what you buy if you want to save money. The food you throw away is money down the drain. If you still bought too much, then try making stock out of vegetables that are starting to get limp. If your meat is going to go bad, then freeze it. If your fruit is going bad, then try dehydrating it so that it keeps for a little while longer or make a homemade jam with natural sweeteners.

## Don't Shop Hungry

Planning your grocery shopping is important because if you can stay within your budget while going paleo, you're more likely to stick to it as a lifestyle change. Make sure that you never go shopping when you're hungry. If you shop on an empty stomach, you're more likely to make decisions based on that hunger than based on need. You may even give into the temptation of buying non-paleo foods.

## Not a Planner?

Being flexible is great too! Even if you make a plan, be flexible if you want to succeed. If you don't have a plan, just plan the amount of money you want to spend and eat before you go. Not planning each and every detail can even help you to save money in the long run because you can shop by sales! Buying in bulk, such as with versatile foods, can help to make your meals budget friendly too. Just never buy more than you can use.

# Chapter 7: Some Success Strategies

Now that you know how a paleo diet works, you're able to start your paleo journey.  Every diet comes with its own challenges, and a paleo diet is no different.

## Withdrawals

When you stop giving your body something that it's used to having, you're going to go through withdrawals. So you'll need to prepare for reduced energy levels, mood swings, cravings, and other withdrawal issues.

## Some Financial Challenges

Shopping for a paleo diet isn't always easy for everyone. You will spend more money when shopping for groceries at first, and shopping won't be as easy since you can't choose from anything on the shelf. Just be aware of the issue and explore your options.

## Exercise is Necessary

No diet is a miracle diet, and you'll need to increase your physical activity if you want the best results. You can't live on junk, fast food, and coffee, especially without exercise. You should schedule time to exercise each and every day.

## Free-Range, Grass-fed & Organic

There is an emphasis on organic products when you're eating a paleo diet. If you can't go full paleo for now, then try to incorporate a paleo lifestyle little by little.

Don't beat yourself up over not being able afford a paleo diet right away or make all of the changes at once. Just try to meet the requirements you can, and always work on incorporating more and more of a paleo diet into your everyday life.

## Maximizing Your Chances

The bottom line is that not every diet will work for every single person. A paleo diet meal plan may work for you, but it may not be suitable for your day to day life regardless of the benefits that it has. Even if you can't use the full diet, trying to become paleo friendly will improve your health. By starting with little changes you maximize your chances of being able to stick with the changes you do implement.

## Using the 80/20 Approach

Few people can be as strict as they actually need to at the beginning of their paleo journey. If you don't cheat with one thing, it's often another. For example, you may be able to give up sweets, but it may be hard to give up those cocktails. You may be able start with grass-fed meat, but your coffee may be a weak spot. To succeed, try not to fall of the wagon. This is where the 80/20 approach comes in handy. When applied to food, you're eating paleo eighty percent of the time and twenty percent of the time you're enjoying non-paleo foods. This allows for fewer restrictions, allowing you to indulge on forbidden food on occasion.

## Free Days & Cheat Days

You can't eat paleo and remain physically inactive. You have to increase your activity, so eighty percent of the time you'll want to be active, but twenty percent of the time you can chill out. However, the trick is scheduling activity-free days so that you don't hit a slump.

# Chapter 8: Possible Side Effects

We've briefly talked about withdrawals already, but you'll want to know of a few other side affects you may experience.


## A Low Carb "Flu"

When your body is used to carbs, it's going to go through withdrawals when you aren't giving it those carbs anymore. You'll feel tired, aggravated, and unsteady for a while when you give up carbs from your diet such as starches, grains and legumes. Even if you can eat enough plant based carbs, it may be too much for your body if you ate a lot of pasta, rice, lentils and bread before.

The low carb flu usually ends after three to four weeks, so if you can tough it out, you'll notice it gets a little better. After three to four weeks your body is used to burning the fat as fuel, so the flu symptoms simply go away. If you want to reduce the risk of getting the low carb flu, you'll want to start to slowly cut own your carbs instead of drastically cutting them out of your diet. If you gradually introduce your body to less and less carbs, it can get used to the change.


## Bad Breath

Don't get a paleo diet mixed up with the ketogenic diet. The ketogenic diet is meant to keep you in the state of ketosis, but a paleo diet is just meant to trigger this state. Still, a paleo diet will have you enter into a state of ketosis, and acetone is an offshoot which has a scent to it. How bad your breath is will depend on how much physical activity you have and your personal body as well. You can chew on fresh herbs or just keep mouthwash with you. Eventually, your body will even out and the bad breath should go away.

## Experiencing Cravings

When you're changing diets, you're going to long for food that you can't have. Cravings are only natural. When your body has shifted, the cravings will lesson, and you can find paleo friendly substitutions for what you're craving too. Remember the 80/20 rule, and it'll be easier to stick with a paleo diet.

## Too Much Protein

A paleo diet embraces different proteins from eggs, fish, poultry and meat in general. However, too much protein can be a bad thing. The poultry, red meat, and eggs can be full of cholesterol and saturated fat, so you need to be careful. Too much animal protein will leave to harmful LDL cholesterol levels, the decrease of good HDL cholesterol, and increase your risk of heart disease. Make sure that you keep your diet balanced with fruits and vegetables to avoid this!

# Chapter 9: Paleo Diet Types

One of the main reasons that a paleo diet is so popular is because it can be tailored to your health requirements as well as conditions. It can take into account your religious practices, food allergies, and moral restraints. You can tailor a paleo diet for your nutritional requirements for each point of your life, which often leads to success. Here are a few standard paleo diet types below so that you can pick the one that works best for you!

## The Basic Paleo Diet

This is considered to be the traditional paleo diet where there is no soy, dairy, grains, refined foods or processed foods. There is no bogus fats, so essentially the diet is stricter. There is no room for cheat days or exceptions in this version of a paleo diet.

## Going with the 80/20 Paleo Diet

Most people go with this type of paleo diet because it allows for mistakes, making it easier to stick with. After all, you can have the foods you love and miss twenty percent of the time. this is great for people who have kids, enjoy going out with friends, or have family dinners.

## The Auto-Immune Paleo Diet

Also known as AIP, this is an adaptation of a paleo diet that is free of foods that cause inflammatory reactions. This type of paleo is commonly used by people who have persistent auto-immune conditions that they need to account for. This includes but is not limited to multiple sclerosis, lupus eczema, fibromyalgia, rheumatoid arthritis, Crohn's disease and IBS. This version of a paleo diet also avoids nightshades which includes eggplants, peppers, potatoes and tomatoes. The auto-immune paleo diet also avoids eggs, nuts and seeds. This type of paleo diet can also be used by those that suffer from poor digestion or intestinal irritation.

## Ketogenic Paleo Diet

If someone has an enormous amount of weight that they want to shed, diabetes they wish to control, or wish to build an excessive amount of muscle, then the ketogenic paleo diet may be for them. It can also be used to treat epilepsy when talked about with your doctor.

## The "Pegan" Paleo Diet

The combination of a paleo and vegan diet can often be referred to as the pegan diet. It's exactly what it sounds like too! It's a paleo diet that's also vegan friendly. This diet is not recommended if you have an auto-immune disease or suffer from persistent health issues.

# Paleo Diet Benefits

Never forget that a paleo diet comes with various benefits which are listed below! There are many reasons to go paleo today.

## Reduced Inflammation

Inflammation is caused by damage to the lining of your digestive system. Chronic inflammation can cause increased sensitivity in your immune system as well. It'll also trigger allergies, asthma, and other health issues that can be eliminated with a paleo diet. This is because a paleo diet cuts out the main culprits of inflammation which is alcohol, sugar, gluten and dairy.

## Less Cravings

This one may throw you for a loop since a paleo diet can actually cause cravings when you first start. However, once you get past a paleo flu, you'll experience less cravings overall since your body will be getting exactly what it needs to function. Due to the intake of healthy fats and proteins, you'll feel more sated with a paleo diet.

## Increased Gut Health

Gut health is important to your overall health, and this is another way that a paleo diet comes in handy. Your gut has gut flora, also known as trillions of microbes, which help you to synthesize vitamins, boost your immune system, regulate metabolism, and digest your food. A paleo diet contributes to a healthier gut because the food promotes the restoration of your gut flora.

## Restful Sleep

Paleo is good for your mind, body and soul, and with a body that's properly fueled, you're likely to sleep smarter. When you feel energized during the day, get all the nutrition that you need, and exercise moderately, you'll find that restful sleep comes naturally. Many people that have switched to a paleo diet say they even fall asleep faster. With a paleo diet, your body is also under less stress because it's no longer dealing with spikes in your blood sugar, gastrointestinal distress, or dealing with excessive caffeine before bed.

## Healthy Headspace

Stress is one of the main culprits of overeating, bad sleep, and bad lifestyle habits. When you start a paleo diet, you're shifting towards a better head space. Better nutrition will give you more mental clarity, more energy, and the ability to become more physically fit.

## Zero Calorie Counting

Many people don't want to have to count every calorie that they put into their body, and you don't have to with a paleo diet. You can eat as much as you need or want to get food as long as you're eating the right things. Whole, natural foods will keep you feeling satisfied. Of course, if you're looking for a specific result, you may want to count the calories still. It all depends on what you're trying to do with a paleo diet, but it is not necessary for gradual weight loss.

## Energized without Caffeine

You already know that having more energy can improve your life. It's why so many people suck down energy drink after energy drink, but there will be no more need for that once you get used to a paleo diet. Natural energy is the best kind, and that's exactly what a paleo diet provides you.

# Recipes to Start With

You'll need some easy paleo recipes to get you started on the right track. There's no reason that eating paleo has to be hard. Give your body what it needs while you give your taste buds what they want.


## Eggs & Tomato Breakfast

This easy paleo dish will be on your favorite ways to start the day in no time! It'll delight your taste buds and leave you feeling full and satisfied.

**Serves:** 2

**Time:** 15 Minutes

**Ingredients:**

- 2 Eggs, Medium
- 2 Tomatoes, Large
- Sea Salt & Black Pepper to Taste
- 1 Teaspoon Parsley, Chopped Fine

**Directions:**

1. Start by cutting off the tops of your tomatoes, scooping the flesh out before lining them on a prepared baking sheet.
2. Start by cracking an egg in each of your tomatoes, and then sprinkle your eggs with sea salt and black pepper.
3. Set your oven to 350 and allow it to preheat before placing your tomatoes in the oven. Bake for a half hour.
4. Remove your tomatoes from the oven, and then season with sea salt, pepper, and parsley.
5. Serve while still warm.

**Nutrition Facts:**

**Calories:** 180

**Fat:** 10 Grams

**Protein:** 14 Grams

# Breakfast Burrito

Just because you can't have tortillas anymore, doesn't mean you can't have a burrito to take on the go.

**Serves:** 1

**Time:** 10 Minutes

**Ingredients:**

- 2 Slices Ham, Medium thickness
- 2 Eggs, Large
- ¼ Cup Chopped Spinach
- 1 Teaspoon Olive Oil
- Salsa to Garnish
- Cilantro to Garnish
- Guacamole to Garnish

**Directions:**

1. Sauté your spinach in your olive oil over medium heat. It should take about two minutes for your spinach to wilt.
2. Whisk your eggs, pouring them over your vegetables.
3. Scramble the mixture with your spatula, and then cook until your eggs are set.
4. Roll your eggs and spinach mixture up in your ham, and then return it back to the skillet.
5. Grill for about half a minute. It should brown slightly.
6. Unroll, and garnish with your toppings before rolling it back up.

**Nutrition Information:**

**Calories:** 394

**Fat:** 25 Grams

**Protein:** 21 Grams

## Easy Breakfast Muffins

Muffins are easy to make in advance when you deal with a busy lifestyle, which is why this paleo friendly breakfast muffin recipe can come in handy.

**Serves:** 4

**Time:** 40 Minutes

**Ingredients:**

- 1 Cup Kale, Fresh & Chopped Coarse
- ½ Cup Almond Milk, Unsweetened
- ¼ Cup Chives, Fresh & Chopped Fine
- 6 Eggs, Medium
- Sea Salt & Black Pepper to Taste
- Coconut Oil for Greasing

**Directions:**

1. Start by taking out a bowl, mixing your kale, chives and eggs together. Make sure to whisk well before continuing.
2. Add in your sea salt and black pepper to taste before adding in your almond milk. Stir until well incorporated.
3. Grease eight muffin tins with your coconut oil, and then divide the batter equally.
4. Preheat your oven to 350, and then bake for a half hour after it's preheated.
5. Allow them to cool down before transferring your muffins onto a plate to serve or store them for later.
6. You can serve them cool or warm!

**Nutrition Facts:**

**Calories:** 100

**Fat:** 5 Grams

**Protein:** 14 Grams

## Simple Kale Omelet

Sometimes when you're just starting out on a diet, you'll want to start with the basics.

**Serves:** 1

**Time:** 10 Minutes

**Ingredients:**

- 3 Eggs
- 1 Tablespoons Chives, Fresh & Chopped Fine
- 1 Tablespoon Butter
- 1 Cup Kale, Chopped
- Sea Salt & Black Pepper to Taste

**Directions:**

1. Heat your butter in a frying pan over medium heat, and then add in your kale once it's hot. Cook for five minutes or until soft.
2. Beat your eggs in a bowl, adding in your sea salt, pepper and chives. Mix well.
3. Add your eggs into your pan, and then swirl to spread evenly.
4. Turn your heat to low, and then fold before serving.

**Nutrition Facts:**

**Calories:** 187.7

**Fat:** 13.5 Grams

**Protein:** 12.3 Grams

# Strawberry & Mint Breakfast Salad

Though this salad is a great way to start the day, that doesn't mean you have to make it in the morning. You can make it the night before and enjoy well chilled before starting your daily routine.

**Serves:** 1

**Time:** 10 Minutes

**Ingredients:**

- 2 Cups Strawberries, Fresh & Chopped
- 2 Cups Cucumber, Skinned & Chopped
- ½ Cup Mint, Fresh & Chopped
- 2 Tablespoons Olive Oil
- 1 Tablespoon Lemon Juice, Fresh
- Pinch Sea Salt

**Directions:**

1. Skin your cucumbers before chopping them. Chop your into and strawberries as well.
2. Add all of your ingredients to a bowl, tossing to serve. You can serve either room temperature or chilled.

**Nutrition Facts:**

**Calories:** 70

**Fat:** 1 Gram

**Protein:** 0 Grams

## Easy Banana Pancakes

By making your pancakes with bananas, you're making an easy paleo friendly breakfast that you're sure to enjoy. The best part is that they're easy to make and only take a half hour to make!

**Serves:** 2

**Time:** 30 Minutes

**Ingredients:**

- 4 Eggs, Large
- 2 Bananas, Ripe, Peeled & Chopped
- ¼ Teaspoon Baking Powder
- Coconut Oil, Melted

**Directions:**

1. Mix your bananas and eggs together before adding in your sea salt and baking powder. Make sure to whisk well.
2. Transfer your mixture to a blender or food processor, blending until smooth. This will be your batter, so you don't want any lumps!
3. Place a skillet over medium-high heat and add in your coconut oil. Wait until your oil has heated up.
4. Pour some of your batter in, spreading it into a circle. Cook for one minute per side.
5. Continue until you've used all of your batter, and then serve warm! It's best to top with honey as a sweetener. Remember that most syrups are not paleo friendly.

**Nutrition Facts:**

**Calories:** 120

**Fat:** 2 Grams

**Protein:** 4 Grams

## Plantain Based Pancakes

This plantain pancake recipe is perfect if you have a busy morning alone. It makes just enough for one person, looks excellent, and tastes even better.

**Serves:** 1

**Time:** 20 Minutes

**Ingredients:**

- ¼ Cup Coconut Water
- ¼ cup Coconut Flour
- 3 Eggs, Large
- ½ Plantain, Ripe, Peeled & Chopped
- ¼ Teaspoon Cream of Tartar
- ¼ Teaspoon Baking Soda
- ¼ Teaspoon Chai Spice
- 1 Teaspoon Coconut Oil, Melted
- A Pinch Sea Salt
- 1 Tablespoon Coconut Shavings, Toasted for Garnish
- 1 Tablespoon Coconut Milk for Garnish

**Directions:**

1. Start by placing your eggs, sea salt, coconut water, coconut flour, cream of tartar, plantain, chai spice, and baking soda in a food processor. Pulse until it's well combined.
2. Place a skillet over medium heat, adding in your coconut oil. Once it's heated up add ¼ cup of your batter, spreading it evenly.
3. Cook until it becomes a golden brown color, flipping your pancake and cooking on the next side. It will take one to two minutes per side.
4. Serve your pancakes with coconut milk and shaved coconut.

**Nutrition Facts:**

**Calories:** 372

**Fat:** 17 Grams

**Protein:** 23 Grams

## Easy Sweet Potato Waffles

You need very few ingredients for these easy paleo friendly waffles. Just follow the simple directions below and you'll be enjoying naturally sweet waffles in no time at all!

**Serves:** 4

**Time:** 30 Minutes

**Ingredients:**

- 2 Sweet Potatoes, Medium, Peeled & Finely Grated
- 3 Eggs, Large
- 1 Teaspoon Cinnamon Powder
- 2 Tablespoons Coconut Oil, Melted
- ½ Teaspoon Nutmeg, Ground
- Natural Applesauce for Garnish

**Directions:**

1. Get out a bowl, mixing your sweet potatoes, coconut oil, eggs, nutmeg and cinnamon together. Make sure that your batter is whisked well.
2. Heat up a waffle iron, and then cook your waffles like you normally would.
3. Serve warm and garnished with natural applesauce or honey. Some people even enjoy both!

**Nutrition Facts:**

**Calories:** 227

**Fat:** 6 Grams

**Protein:** 6 Grams

# Granola Toasting Bread

You may not be able to have bread on a paleo diet, but you can use this delicious bread substitute with a paleo friendly jam for breakfast! You can also use it for sandwiches and more.

**Serves:** 4

**Time:** 50 Minutes

**Ingredients:**

- ¾ Cup Dried Apricots, Chopped
- ¾ Cup Pistachios, Shelled
- 2 Cups Old Fashioned Rolled Oats, Gluten Free
- ½ Cup Sunflower Seeds
- ¾ Cup Shredded Coconut, Unsweetened
- ½ Cup Pepitas
- ½ Cup Flax Seeds, Whole
- 1/3 Cup Psyllium Husks
- 3 Tablespoons Chia Seeds
- 1 Teaspoon Cinnamon
- 2 Teaspoon Sea Salt, Fine
- 2 ½ Cups Water
- 1/8 Teaspoon Cardamom
- 1 Teaspoon Vanilla Extract, Pure
- ¼ Cup Olive Oil
- ¼ Cup Maple Syrup, Pure

**Directions:**

1. Combine your oats, pistachios, apricots, shredded coconut, sunflower seeds, pepitas, whole flax seeds, psyllium husks, chia seeds, sea salt, cardamom and cinnamon together in a bowl. Make sure to mix well.

2.  In a different bowl combine all of your remaining ingredients.

3.  Mix your wet ingredients and your dry ingredients together, whisking until well combined.

4.  Grease a loaf pan before pouring in your batter. Chill for two hours, and then bake at 400 for an hour and a half.

**Nutrition Facts:**

**Calories:** 189

**Fat:** 12.6 Grams

**Protein:** 4.9 Grams

# Roasted Mushrooms & Herbs

This is another great paleo recipe that's great for lunch! These mushrooms are filling and packed full of flavor too.

**Serves:** 6

**Time:** 55 Minutes

**Ingredients:**

- ¼ Cup Olive Oil
- ½ Cup Loosely Packed Herbs, Fresh & Blended (Marjoram, Flat Leaf Parsley, Chives, & Thyme Minced)
- Sea Salt & Black Pepper to Taste
- ¼ lb. Shiitake Mushrooms, Washed & Sliced
- ¾ lb. Cremini Mushrooms, Washed & Sliced

**Directions:**

1. Start by turning your oven to 475, and prepare a baking sheet for your mushrooms. Lay out your mushrooms, roasting for twenty minutes. Flip your mushrooms and cook for another ten minutes.
2. Allow your mushrooms to cool before mixing them with your remaining ingredients.
3. Serve warm.


**Nutrition Facts:**

**Calories:** 299

**Fat:** 27.5 Grams

**Protein:** 5.9 Grams

# Zucchini & Chorizo

Zucchini has many health benefits, including maintaining eye health, providing potassium, improving digestion, and it even has anti-inflammatory properties. It's even packed with antioxidants, low in calories, a great source of B vitamins, and a wonderful source of vitamin C.

**Serves:** 4

**Time:** 35 Minutes

**Ingredients:**

- 1 Teaspoon Olive Oil
- 1 Lime, Juiced & Zested
- ½ Cup Packed Cilantro, Chopped Rough
- 4 Medium Zucchini, Cubed in ¾ Inch Pieces
- 4 Ounces Spanish Chorizo, Cubed in 1/3 Inch Pieces
- Sea Salt to Taste

**Directions:**

1. Start by placing a skillet over medium-high heat, browning it for four to five minutes. Once browned, place your chorizo in a bowl.
2. In another pan place the rest of your ingredients, cooking for ten to twelve minutes. Your vegetables should become tender. Stir often to avoid burning.
3. Add all of your ingredients together, mixing well before serving while still warm.

**Nutrition Facts:**

**Calories:** 177

**Fat:** 12.6 Grams

**Protein:** 9.4 Grams

## Onion & Citrus Salad

This combination may sound a bit strange at first, but once you try it you'll be hooked! This salad is refreshing and easy to make.

**Serves:** 2

**Time:** 5 Minutes

**Ingredients:**

- ¼ Teaspoon Cumin Seeds, Toasted & Crushed
- 1 Tablespoon Olive Oil
- Sea Salt to Taste
- 1/8 Cup Mint Leaves, Fresh
- 6 Black Olives, Pitted
- 1 Small Onion, Sliced Thin
- 2 Oranges, Peeled, Sliced & Seeded
- 1 Small Grapefruit, Peeled, Sliced & Seeded

**Directions:**

1. Toss everything in a bowl, seasoning with your salt before serving.

**Nutrition Facts:**

**Calories:** 294

**Fat:** 7.2 Grams

**Protein:** 3 Grams

# Simple Beef Stew

You may have to give up canned soup because they aren't paleo friendly, but you can still make a healthy stew that your family is sure to enjoy without breaking your diet.

**Serves:** 6

**Time:** 1 Hour 10 Minutes

**Ingredients:**

- 1 lb. Lean, Grass-fed Beef, Ground
- 1 lb. Grass-fed Sausage, Sliced
- 4 Cups Beef Stock, Low Sodium
- 30 Ounces Tomatoes, Canned & Diced
- 3 Zucchinis, Chopped
- 1 Green Bell Pepper, Chopped
- 1 Cup Celery, Chopped
- 1 Teaspoon Italian Seasoning, Homemade
- ½ Yellow Onion, Diced
- ½ Teaspoon Oregano, Dried
- ½ Teaspoon Basil, Dried
- ¼ Teaspoon Garlic Powder
- Sea Salt & Black Pepper to Taste

**Directions:**

1. Place your meat into a pot, cooking until it browns and drain away your excess fat.
2. Add in all of your other ingredients, bringing the mixture to a boil. Stir well!
3. Reduce the heat to medium-low, allowing your stew to simmer for an hour before serving warm.

**Nutrition Facts:**

**Calories:** 370

**Fat:** 17 Grams

**Protein:** 25 Grams

# Root Based Soup

Root vegetables are fantastic and usually cheap too. They're easy to make into a soup, and perfect for winter!

**Serves:** 8

**Time:** 1 Hour 40 minutes

**Ingredients:**

- 2 Tablespoons Butter, Unsalted
- 5 Carrots, Chopped
- 1 Sweet Onion, Chopped
- 3 Parsnips, Chopped
- 3 Beets, Chopped
- 3 Bacon Slices
- 1 Quart Chicken Stock, Low Sodium
- Sea Salt & Black Pepper to Taste
- 2 Quarts Water, Natural
- ½ Teaspoon Chili Flakes
- ½ Tablespoon Thyme, Dried
- ½ Tablespoon Rosemary, Dried

**Directions:**

1. Start by heating up a Dutch oven over medium-high heat and add in your butter. Once your butter is hot, then add in your onion. Stir and cook for five minutes or until your onion is tender.
2. Add in your parsnips, beets, bacon, chicken stock, water and carrots. Stir to combine.
3. Season with your sea salt and black pepper to taste before adding your rosemary, thyme, and chili flakes, and stir again.
4. Bring your mixture to a boil before reducing it to medium-low heat.

5. Allow the mixture to simmer for an hour and a half.

6. Serve warm.

**Nutrition Facts:**

**Calories:** 180

**Fat:** 2 Grams

**Protein:** 3.5 Grams

## Shrimp Stuffed Avocado & Spring Greens

Avocado is a great source of healthy fats, which balances out the high cholesterol in the shrimp. You'll find that this recipe is full of calcium too!

**Serves:** 4

**Time:** 20 Minutes

**Ingredients:**

- 1 Cup Shrimp, Cooked & Small
- 1 Mango, Ripe & Diced
- ¼ Teaspoon Chili Flakes, Dried
- 1 Lime, Juiced & Zested
- 1/8 Cup Cilantro, Chopped Fine
- Sea Salt & Black Pepper to Taste
- 2 Avocados, Halved & Pitted
- 1 Tablespoon Olive Oil
- ¼ Cup Herb Salad Greens for Serving

**Directions:**

1. Start by tossing your shrimp, mango, chili flakes, cilantro, lime, sea salt, and pepper together. Make sure to mix well.
2. Scoop the mixture into your avocado before drizzling the olive oil over it. Top with your herbs before serving.

**Nutrition Facts:**

**Calories:** 31

**Fat:** 3.4 Grams

**Protein:** 0.2 Grams

# Paleo Chicken Soup

Everyone loves chicken soup. For some people, it's something to eat when they're sick, and for others it's just a favorite that reminds them of home. No matter why you like it, you'll find that there is a paleo version that you can enjoy! Just follow the recipe below.

**Serves:** 6

**Time:** 45 Minutes

**Ingredients:**

- 2 Celery Stalks, Chopped
- 2 Carrots, Chopped
- ½ Cup Coconut Oil, Melted
- 6 Cups Chicken Broth, Low Sodium
- ½ Cup Arrowroot Powder
- 1 Teaspoon Parsley, Dried
- ½ Cup Water
- 1-2 Bay Leaves
- Sea Salt & Black Pepper to Taste
- ½ Teaspoon Thyme, Dried
- 1 ½ Cups Coconut Milk, Unsweetened
- 3 Cups Chicken Breast, Cooked & Diced

**Directions:**

1. Start by getting out a heavy bottomed soup pot, placing your coconut oil inside. Place your pot over medium-high heat.
2. Add in your celery and carrots, cooking for ten minutes. Your vegetables should become tender, but stir frequently to avoid burning.
3. Dump in your chicken broth, and then bring your mixture to a boil.

4. Take a bowl, mixing your arrowroot powder with ½ cup of water, whisking to combine.

5. Add your arrowroot mixture to your soup, mixing well before seasoning with your sea salt and pepper.

6. Stir, and then add in your parsley, bay leaves, and thyme.

7. Stir again before adding in your coconut milk and chicken, cooking for one to two more minutes. Turn off the heat.

8. Serve warm.

**Nutrition Facts:**

**Calories:** 412

**Fat:** 31 Grams

**Protein:** 27 Grams

# Garlic & Lemon Soup

While soup is easy to make, you don't want to get bored with it too quickly! That's where this strange but delicious soup comes in handy.

**Serves:** 4

**Time:** 30 Minutes

**Ingredients:**

- 6 Cups Shellfish Stock
- 1 Tablespoon Garlic, Minced Fine
- 1 Tablespoon Ghee
- 2 Eggs, Large
- ½ Cup Lemon Juice, Fresh
- Sea Salt & White Pepper to Taste
- 1 Tablespoon Arrowroot Powder
- Cilantro, Finely Chopped for Garnish

**Directions:**

1. Start by placing a heavy bottomed saucepan over medium-high heat and adding in your ghee.
2. Once your ghee is warm, add in your garlic. Cook while stirring for two minutes, making sure that your garlic doesn't burn. It should become fragrant.
3. Add your stock, reserving a half a cup for later, and bring your garlic and stock to a simmer.
4. In a bowl, mix your eggs, sea salt, white pepper, reserved stock, and lemon juice together. Make sure to whisk until fully combined.
5. Pour your egg mixture into your soup, stirring again until well combined. Allow it to cook for four to five minutes.
6. Ladle into soup bowls while it's warm, and serve with your chopped cilantro.

**Nutrition Facts:**

**Calories:** 135

**Fat:** 3 Grams

**Protein:** 8 Grams

# Salmon cakes

These are great to have on their own as a snack, for lunch, or to go with your paleo friendly diner. They're great for your heart and brain because they're loaded with healthy omega-3.

**Serves:** 3

**Time:** 10 Minutes

**Ingredients:**

- 1 Can Boneless & Skinless Salmon
- ½ Onion, Peeled & Diced
- 1 Tablespoon Dried Dill
- 1 ½ Tablespoons Coconut Flour
- 1 Teaspoon Lemon Pepper
- 3 Tablespoons Coconut Oil
- ¼ Teaspoon Sea Salt, Fine
- 1 Stalk Celery, Diced

**Directions:**

1. Start by breaking your salmon up with a fork, and then add in your spices, celery, and diced onion. Mix, and then add in your coconut flour. You'll want to make sure it's thoroughly combined.
2. Add in your eggs, mixing again.
3. Puta skillet over medium heat with your coconut oil into it. Allow for the mixture to heat up while you divide your salmon mixture into five two inch wide pieces.
4. Add your patties to the heated oil, cooking for two to three minutes per side. Your patties should be lightly browned.

**Nutrition Facts:**

**Calories:** 198.8

**Fat:** 9.4 Grams

**Protein:** 24.4 Grams

# Cabbage & Beef Bowl

This cabbage and beef bowl is paleo friendly and the perfect one dish meal.

**Serves:** 4

**Time:** 10 Minutes

**Ingredients:**

- 1 lb. Ground Beef
- 1 Carrot, Grated
- 5 Cups Napa Cabbage, Sliced Thin
- 2 Tablespoons Coconut Oil
- 1 Onion, Chopped
- Sea Salt & Black Pepper to Taste

**Directions:**

1. Start by heating a skillet over medium heat before adding in your coconut oil. Once your oil is hot, add in your ground beef and onion.
2. Cook while stirring occasionally until your beef is cooked all the way through, and your onion should be tender and translucent. Add in your cabbage and carrots, sating until softened.
3. Remove from heat, drizzling with hot sauce if desired before serving.


**Nutrition Facts:**

**Calories:** 39.7

**Fat:** 2.7 Gras

**Protein:** 12.3 Grams

# Blackened Cajun Salmon

When people imagine salmon, they often don't imagine a taste of the south, which is exactly what you get with this blackened Cajun salmon recipe.

**Serves:** 2

**Time:** 10 Minutes

**Ingredients:**

- 2 Salmon Fillets, 6 Ounces Each
- 1 Tablespoon Coconut Oil
- 1 Tablespoon Cilantro, Fresh & Chopped

**Cajun Rub:**

- ¼ Teaspoon Garlic Powder
- ¼ Teaspoon Onion Powder
- ¼ Teaspoon Sea Salt, Fine
- 1/8 Teaspoon Ground Black Pepper
- ¼ Teaspoon Cayenne Pepper
- ½ Teaspoon Thyme, Dried
- ½ Teaspoon Oregano, Dried
- 1 Teaspoon Smoked Paprika

**Directions:**

1. Stir all of your rub ingredients except your salmon and cilantro in a bowl before rubbing the mixture over your salmon. Make sure that you're rubbing the mixture over the skinless side.
2. Melt your coconut oil in a skillet over medium heat, placing your salmon with the skin side facing upward.
3. Sear for four minutes, and it should be brown.
4. Flip it over, cooking for another four minutes.

5. Garnish with cilantro before serving.

**Nutrition Facts:**

**Calories:** 430

**Fat:** 25 Grams

**Protein:** 45 Grams

# Brussel Slaw

This is great at a lunch or a side dish! It even has protein due to the bacon too.

**Serves:** 4

**Time:** 10 Minutes

**Ingredients:**

- 2 Package Brussel Sprouts, Shredded
- 1 Package Bacon
- ½ Sweet Onion, Chopped
- 1 Tablespoon Balsamic Vinegar
- Sea Salt & Black Pepper to Taste

**Directions:**

1. Slice your onion and then add it to your skillet along with your bacon.
2. Cook your bacon and onion for three to four minutes. Your bacon should be crispy and your onions tender.
3. Add in your balsamic vinegar, deglazing the pan, and then add in your shredded Brussel sprouts. Mix everything together.
4. Cover the pan and allow it to steam for two to three minutes.
5. Season with salt and pepper before serving.

**Nutrition Facts:**

**Calories:** 176.5

**Fat:** 11.9 Grams

**Protein:** 6.6 Grams

# Avocado & Watermelon Soup

With its bright color, creamy texture, and unique taste, this is another paleo soup recipe you're sure to enjoy!

**Serves:** 3

**Time:** 10 Minutes

**Ingredients:**

- 1 Avocado, Pitted, Peeled & Chopped
- 1 Cucumber, Cut
- ½ Cup Baby Spinach
- 1 ½ Cups Watermelon, Chopped
- ¼ Cup Cilantro, Chopped Rough
- ½ Cup Coconut Aminos
- ½ cup Lime Juice, Fresh
- 2 Lemons, Juiced

**Directions:**

1. Blend all ingredients together in a high speed blender or food processor. Blend until completely smooth.
2. Transfer to soup bowls and serve room temperature or chilled.

**Nutrition Facts:**

**Calories:** 100

**Fat:** 7 Grams

**Protein:** 2.3 Grams

## Guacamole Salad

This is the perfect recipe if you need a paleo meal on the go. It's easy to make in advance and take with you without losing its flavor.

**Serves:** 4

**Time:** 10 Minutes

**Ingredients:**

- 1 Clove Garlic, Minced
- Sea Salt & Black Pepper to Taste
- ¼ cup Lime Juice, Fresh
- 2 Avocadoes, Pitted & Diced
- 3 Tablespoons Olive Oil
- 1 Pint Cherry Tomatoes, Halved
- ¼ Red Onion, Diced Fine
- ¼ Cup Cilantro, Fresh & Chopped

**Directions:**

1. Mix your garlic, pepper and lime juice together.
2. Whisk your olive oil in, and then add in your avocado, cilantro, tomatoes and onion.
3. Adjust your pepper and sea salt to taste, and serve room temperature or chilled.

**Nutrition Facts:**

**Calories:** 111.3

**Fat:** 9 Grams

**Protein:** 1.7 Grams

# Bok Choy & Pumpkin

When you're going paleo, you'll want to keep your diet interesting. Most people n
ever get the chance to cook with bok choy, but it's a delicious Asian vegetable
that's sure to bring a little extra flavor to your table.

**Serves:** 4

**Time:** 25 Minutes

**Ingredients:**

- 2 Teaspoons Sesame Oil
- 3 Tablespoons Coconut Aminos
- 1 Inch Ginger, Peeled & Grated
- 2 Tablespoons Olive Oil
- ¼ Teaspoon Red Pepper Flakes
- 4 Bok Choy Heads, Quartered
- 3 Garlic Cloves, Minced
- 1 Small Pumpkin, Peeled, Seeded & Sliced Thin
- 1 Tablespoon Sesame Seeds, Toasted

**Directions:**

1. Start by placing a pan over medium heat, adding in your olive oil and sesame seeds. Stir well before adding in your coconut aminos, pepper flakes, ginger, and garlic. Stir well, cooking for one minute before removing it from heat.
2. Take another pan, adding water, and bringing it to a simmer over medium-high heat. Add in your pumpkin pieces, covering the pan and cooking for ten minutes.
3. Drain your pumpkin slices, transferring them to a plate to cool.
4. Add your bok choy to your remaining water, heating it over medium-high heat again. Cover, cooking for another five minutes.

5. Drain, and then add them to the platter that has your pumpkins.
6. Add in your sesame oil mix from the pan, and then toss your sesame seeds on top.
7. Serve warm.

**Nutrition Facts:**

**Calories:** 160

**Fat:** 2 Grams

**Protein:** 5 Grams

## Coconut & Lamb Stew

This stew recipe comes all the way from India, bringing a new taste to your table. One of the main ways people stick to a new diet is by making it exciting and trying new things, which is where this easy stew recipe comes in handy.

**Serves:** 4

**Time:** 2 Hours 5 Minutes

**Ingredients:**

- 1 Tablespoon Coconut Oil, Melted
- 1 ½ lbs. Lamb Meat, Grass-fed & Diced
- ½ Red Chili, Seedless & Chopped
- 1 Brown Onion, Chopped Rough
- 3 Cloves Garlic, Minced Fine
- 2 Celery Stalks, Chopped
- 1 Tablespoon Lemon Juice, Fresh
- 2 ½ Teaspoons Garam Masala Powder
- 1 Teaspoon Fennel Seeds, Whole

- 14 Ounces Coconut Milk, Canned
- 1 ½ Tablespoons Coconut Milk, Unsweetened
- 1 Cup Water
- Sea Salt & Black Pepper to Taste
- 1 ¼ Teaspoons Turmeric, Ground
- 1 ½ Teaspoons Ghee
- Parsley, Chopped Fine for Garnish

**Directions:**

1. Start by heating up a heavy bottomed soup pan over medium-high heat, and then add in your oil.
2. Once your oil is hot, add in your lam, stirring well. Brown your lamb for four minutes. It should have a slight crisp to it.
3. Add in your chili, onion, and celery, cooking for another minute. You'll need to stir so that your ingredients don't stick, and they should become fragrant in this time.
4. Reduce your heat to medium before adding in your ghee, garlic, garam masala, turmeric, and fennel. Cook while stirring for a full minute.
5. Season with your sea salt and black pepper before adding in your coconut milk, water, and tomato paste. Stir your mixture well before bringing it to a boil.
6. Reduce your heat to low, covering your pot.
7. Allow it to simmer for a full hour to get a strong flavor.
8. Add your carrots in, covering again and cooking for another forty minutes. You'll need to stir your soup every once in a while.
9. Add in your lemon juice and parsley before stirring again.
10. Take your soup off of heat and serve warm.

**Nutrition Facts:**

**Calories:** 450

**Fat:** 31 Grams

## Simple Lamb Chops

These lamb chops are seasoned lightly to bring out the taste of your meat, and it's best to pair with any green vegetable or salad.

**Serves:** 2

**Time:** 30 Minutes

**Ingredients:**

- 4 Lamb Chops
- 1 Lemon, Juiced
- 1/8 Cup Olive Oil
- Fresh Thyme to Taste
- Sea Salt to Taste

**Directions:**

1. Place your lamb chops in a baking dish, covering them with your lemon juice. Drizzle your olive oil over them, and then add in your thyme leaves. Cover, and then let them marinate for twenty minutes. You'll need to turn them halfway through.
2. Preheat your top grill over high heat. Lower the heat before adding on your lamb chops, cooking for three minutes per side. Grill your lemons with your lamb chops.
3. Serve while warm, sprinkling more thyme and sea salt over them.

**Nutrition Facts:**

**Calories:** 250.2 Grams

**Fat:** 11 Grams

**Protein:** 47.2 Grams

# Beef Liver & Onions

Beef liver is great for you, and it can taste great too, especially when it's piled with seasoned onions.

**Serves:** 4

**Time:** 20 Minutes

**Ingredients:**

- ¾ lb. Beef Liver, Marinated as Desired & Sliced
- 1 Teaspoon Thyme, Fresh & Chopped
- 1 Teaspoon Sage, Fresh & Chopped
- 3 Tablespoon Lard
- Sea Salt to Taste
- 1 Sweet Onion, Sliced Thin

**Directions:**

1. Melt your lard in a nonstick pan over low heat.
2. Add in your chopped herbs, stirring before adding in your onion. Cook your onion until translucent, which should take about ten minutes.
3. Place your onions to the side, and then increase your heat to medium-high. Add another tablespoon of lard.
4. Add your liver once your lard is hot, sautéing for about three minutes or until browned on one side.
5. Flip your liver, adding your onions back to your pan, and then cook for two more minutes until the inside is pink.

**Nutrition Facts:**

**Calories:** 468

**Fat:** 18.3 Grams

**Protein:** 41 Grams

## Glazed Chicken & Green Beans

This dinner recipe has everything you need to sit down and eat, but it's anything but boring.

**Serves:** 4

**Time:** 30 Minutes

**Ingredients:**

- 6 Tablespoons Chicken Stock, Unsalted
- 1/3 Cup Honey, Raw
- 2 Tablespoons Dark Sesame Oil
- 1 ½ Tablespoons Whole Grain Mustard
- 4 Chicken Breasts, Boneless, Skinless & 6 Ounces
- ¾ Teaspoon Sea Salt, Fine
- ½ Teaspoon Black Pepper
- 2 Teaspoons Sesame Seeds, Toasted
- 8 Ounces Green Beans, Fresh & Trimmed
- 1 Tablespoon Coconut Oil
- 2 Tablespoons Sliced Almonds, Toasted

**Directions:**

1. Start by combining your chicken stock, mustard, a tablespoon of oil, and your honey in your pan. Place the pan over medium heat, whisking as you bring it to a boil. Allow it to cook for ten minutes, but stir occasionally to keep from burning.
2. Place a nonstick skillet over medium heat, adding in another tablespoon of oil. Make sure that your skillet is coated, and then add in your chicken. Sprinkle it liberally with your salt and pepper.
3. Allow your chicken to cook for six minutes, turning halfway through.
4. Add your honey over your chicken, tossing your sesame seeds into coat it.

5. Blanch your green beans, and then cook them for six to eight minutes over medium-high heat with oil. Season with sea salt to taste.

6. Sprinkle your green beans with almonds, and serve with your warm chicken.

**Nutrition Facts:**

**Calories:** 434

**Fat:** 16.8 Grams

**Protein:** 40 Grams

# Homestyle Chili

Chili is a favorite of many, especially during the winter, and with this paleo friendly recipe there's no reason to kiss it goodbye.

**Serves:** 6

**Time:** 1 Hour

**Ingredients:**

- 1 Teaspoon Olive Oil
- 1 ½ lbs. Ground Turkey, Lean
- 3 Cloves Garlic, Minced
- 1 ½ Teaspoon Ground Cumin
- ½ Teaspoon Sea Salt
- 1 Bell Pepper, Chopped
- ¼ Teaspoon Cayenne Pepper
- 15 Ounces Kidney Beans, Canned
- 15 Ounces Tomato Sauce, Canned

**Directions:**

1. Place your oil in a skillet over medium heat, adding in your bell pepper, garlic, turkey and onion. Cook while stirring for ten minutes.
2. Add in your cayenne, cumin, chili powder, and sea salt. Cook and stir for another minute.
3. Add in your tomato sauce and kidney beans, stirring again before bringing it to a boil.
4. Reduce your heat to low, and then allow it to simmer for twenty minutes. It should become thick, but you will need to stir occasionally.
5. Serve while still warm, topped with avocado or diced tomatoes if you want.

**Nutrition Facts:**

**Calories:** 288

**Fat:** 16 Grams

**Protein:** 43 Grams

# Orange Chicken

Orange chicken is a takeout favorite of many, but you can make a paleo version right in your own kitchen.

**Serves:** 2

**Time:** 25 Minutes

**Ingredients:**

- 1 lb. Chicken Thighs, Boneless & Skinless
- 4 Tablespoons Bacon Fat
- Sea Salt & Black Pepper to Taste

**Sauce:**

- 1 Cup Water
- 1 Orange, Zested
- 3 Tablespoons Coconut Aminos
- ½ Cup Orange Juice, Fresh
- Dash Red Pepper Flakes
- 2 Tablespoons Arrowroot Flour
- ½ Teaspoon Ground Ginger

**Directions:**

1. Start by seasoning your chicken liberally with your salt and pepper before placing it to the side.
2. Mix all of your sauce ingredient together in a medium pan over medium heat, stirring frequently. Allow your sauce to thicken before removing it from heat.
3. Heat your bacon fat in a different skillet, adding in your chicken. Allow your chicken to brown on all sides. This should take about seven minutes.

4. Drain your excess fat, and then pour part of your sauce into the pan. Make sure you stir to coat your chicken.

5. Remove your chicken from heat, and pouring the remaining sauce over your steamed vegetables to serve.

**Nutrition Facts:**

**Calories:** 414

**Fat:** 17 Grams

**Protein:** 42 Grams

# Creamy Basil Paleo Chicken

Many people think that when they give up dairy they have to kiss their creamy foods goodbye, but that's not the case with this creamy chicken recipe.

**Serves:** 2

**Time:** 50 Minutes

**Ingredients:**

- 4 Chicken Breasts
- ½ Teaspoon Black Pepper
- 2 Tablespoons Balsamic Vinegar
- ½ Teaspoon Sea Salt, Fine
- 1 Teaspoon Onion Powder
- 1 Teaspoon Italian Seasoning, Homemade
- Olive Oil for Drizzling

**Cream Sauce:**

- 1 Avocado, Ripe
- ½ Cup Basil, Fresh & Chopped
- 1 Tablespoon Lemon Juice, Fresh
- 2 Cloves Garlic, Minced
- ½ Cup Coconut Milk

**Directions:**

1. Start by heating your oven to 375.
2. Get out an eight by eight pan, placing your chicken in it. Top with your balsamic vinegar and olive oil.
3. Mix all of your spices into a bowl, and then place ¼ teaspoon of spice on top of each chicken breast.

4. Bake for forty minutes, and prepare your cream sauce. To do this mix all ingredients in a blender, blending until smooth.

5. Add your coconut milk until you reach the desired consistency, and serve your sauce over your chicken.

**Nutrition Facts:**

**Calories:** 448.7

**Fat:** 28.1 Grams

**Protein:** 43.6 Grams

# French Chicken Stew

This chicken stew will help you to bring a taste of France right to your table.

**Serves:** 4

**Time:** 30 Minutes

**Ingredients:**

- 10 Garlic Cloves, Peeled & Minced
- 30 Black Olives, Pitted
- 2 lbs. Chicken, Cubed
- 2 Cups Chicken Stock, Low Sodium
- 28 Ounces Tomatoes, Canned & Chopped
- 2 Tablespoons Parsley, Fresh & Chopped
- 2 Tablespoons Rosemary, Fresh & Chopped
- 2 Tablespoons Basil, Fresh & Chopped
- Sea Salt & Black Pepper to Taste
- Drizzle of Olive Oil to Serve

**Directions:**

1. Start by placing your pot over medium-high heat, and then add in your olive oil. Add in your chicken before seasoning it with sea salt and pepper. Cook for four minutes, stirring often so that it doesn't stick.
2. Add in your garlic, stirring and cooking for two minutes. Your garlic should brown and become fragrant. If you do not stir often enough it'll burn.
3. Add in your tomatoes, chicken stock, thyme, rosemary, and olives before stirring. Cover your pot, and then turn your oven to 325. Place your stew in an oven safe dish before cooking for an hour.
4. Add in your basil and parsley before mixing and placing it back in the oven. Bake for another forty-five more minutes.

**5.** Allow your stew to cool before serving.

**Nutrition Facts:**

**Calories:** 300

**Fat:** 48 Grams

**Protein:** 61 Grams

## Easy Avocado Boats

Avocado boats are full of healthy omega-3 and other healthy fats. You'll find that they're easy to make too! You'll have a delicious lunch in less than ten minutes, and they're easy to take with you.

**Serves:** 2

**Time:** 10 Minutes

**Ingredients:**

- 1 Lemon, Juiced
- 1 Avocado, Pitted & Halved
- 5 Ounces tuna, Canned, Drained & Flaked
- 1 Tablespoon Yellow Onion, Chopped
- Sea Salt & Black Pepper to Taste

**Directions:**

1. Start by scooping most of your avocado flesh before placing it into a bowl.
2. Add your onion, lemon juice, sea salt and black pepper to the bowl. Stir well.
3. Scoop the mixture into your avocado cups, mixing and serving cooled or room temperature.


**Nutrition Facts:**

**Calories:** 100

**Fat:** 2 Grams

**Protein:** 5 Grams

## Oxtail Stew

Oxtail isn't something most people cook with often, but it's still able to be found in most grocery stores. This paleo diet may be time consuming, but its well worth it!

**Serves:** 8

**Time:** 6 Hours 15 Minutes

**Ingredients:**

- 2 Leeks, Chopped
- 4 Carrots, Chopped
- 4 ½ lbs. Oxtail, Chopped
- Drizzle of Olive Oil
- 1 Tablespoon Olive Oil
- 2 Celery Stalks, Chopped
- 4 Thyme Sprigs, Chopped
- 4 Rosemary Sprigs, Chopped
- 4 Cloves Garlic, Minced
- 4 Bay Leaves
- Sea Salt & Black Pepper to Taste
- 2 Tablespoons All Purpose Flour
- 28 Ounces Plum Tomatoes, Canned & Chopped
- 9 Ounces Dry Red Wine
- 1 Quart Beef Stock, Low Sodium
- Worcestershire Sauce to Taste

**Directions:**

1. Place your oxtail in a roasting pan before seasoning it with your sea salt and black pepper. Drizzle it with olive oil, tossing to coat.
2. Turn your oven to 425 degrees, baking for twenty minutes.

3. Place a pot over medium heat with a tablespoon of olive oil. Allow your oil to heat up, adding in your carrots, celery, and leeks. Stir and cook for about four minutes. Your vegetables should become tender.

4. Add in your rosemary, bay leaves, and thyme before stirring. Allow it to simmer for another twenty minutes while stirring occasionally.

5. Take your oxtail out of the oven, allowing it to cool for a few moments.

6. Add in your flour and cloves to your vegetables, stirring well.

7. Add in your wine, ox tail and tomatoes. You'll want to add in the juices from your oxtail as well. Stir well, and then increase the heat to bring your mixture to a boil.

8. Place it in an oven safe pot, turning your oven down to 325 degrees. Bake for five hours, and then allow it to cool for ten minutes.

9. Discard the bones from your oxtail, returning the meat to the pot. Season with sea salt and pepper before adding in your Worcestershire sauce to taste.

10. Allow it to cool slightly before serving.

**Nutrition Facts:**

**Calories:** 523

**Fat:** 38 Grams

**Protein:** 28 Grams

# Beef Tenderloins with Sauce

These beef tenderloins have a special sauce that bring even more flavor to the dish!

**Serves:** 4

**Time:** 50 Minutes

**Ingredients:**

- 3 lbs. Beef Tenderloin
- Sea Salt & Black Pepper to Taste
- 3 Tablespoons Dijon Mustard
- 3 Tablespoons Balsamic Vinegar
- 1 Tablespoon Coconut Oil

**Sauce:**

- 3 Tablespoons Basil Leaves, Fresh & Chopped
- 1 Lemon, Zested
- ½ Cup Parsley Leaves, Fresh & Chopped
- 2 Cloves Garlic, Chopped Fine
- ¼ Cup Olive Oil
- Sea Salt & Black Pepper to Taste

**Directions:**

1. Start by mixing your mustard and vinegar in a bowl, stirring well. Set it to the side.
2. Season your beef with sea salt and black pepper, and then set it to the side.
3. Place a pan over medium-high heat, adding in your coconut oil. Once your oil is heated, add in your beef, cooking for two minutes per side.
4. Transfer your beef to a prepared baking dish, covering with your mustard sauce, heating your oven to 475. Bake for twenty-five minutes.

5. In a different bowl, mix your basil, parsley, garlic, olive oil, and lemon zest. Season with sea salt and pepper before whisking well.
6. Take your beef tenderloin out, and then set it to the side to cool
7. Serve with your herb sauce and enjoy.

**Nutrition Facts:**

**Calories:** 180

**Fat:** 13 Grams

**Protein:** 7 Grams

# Simple Beef Stir Fry

This simple stir fry is Asian inspired, and it's easy to make too! It's perfect for dinner or lunches.

**Serves:** 4

**Time:** 30 Minutes

**Ingredients:**

- 10 Ounces Asparagus, Sliced
- 10 Ounces Mushrooms, Sliced
- 1 ½ lbs. Beef Steak, Lean & Sliced Thin
- 2 Tablespoons Honey, Raw
- 1/3 Cup Coconut Aminos
- 2 Teaspoons Apple Cider Vinegar, Mother Included
- ½ Teaspoon Ginger, Minced
- 7 Garlic Cloves, Minced
- 1 Chili, Sliced & Seeded
- 1 Tablespoon Coconut Oil, Melted
- Sea Salt & Black Pepper to Taste

**Directions:**

1. Start by mixing your coconut aminos, garlic, honey, vinegar, and ginger in a bowl. Whisk until well combined.
2. Add your water in a pan, placing it over medium-high heat. Once heated, add in your asparagus, cooking for three minutes.
3. Transfer your asparagus into a bowl of ice water, draining and set it to the side.
4. Heat up another pan over medium-high heat, adding in oil. Once your oil is heated, add in your mushrooms, cooing for two minutes on each side. Transfer to a bowl, and set it to the side to cool.

5. Place the pan over high heat again, adding in your meat. Brown for a few minutes before mixing in your chili.

6. Cook for two more minutes before adding in your mushrooms, vinegar sauce and asparagus.

7. Cook for three more minutes before removing it from heat.

8. Serve while still warm!

**Nutrition Facts:**

**Calories:** 165

**Fat:** 7.2 Grams

**Protein:** 18.4 Grams

## BBQ Ribs

Ribs are great to eat for dinner or even take to a pot luck, and they can be paleo too!

**Serves:** 4

**Time:** 3 Hours 5 Minutes

**Ingredients:**

- ½ Tablespoon Onion Powder
- ½ Tablespoon Garlic Powder
- 1 Tablespoon Smoked Paprika
- ½ Teaspoon Cayenne Pepper
- 4 lbs. Baby Back Ribs
- 1 Cup Paleo Friendly BBQ Sauce
- 2 Tablespoons Honey, Raw
- 4 Teaspoon Sriracha
- ¼ Cup Chives, Fresh & Chopped
- ¼ Cup Cilantro, Fresh & Chopped
- ¼ Cup Parsley, Fresh & Chopped
- Sea Salt & Black Pepper to Taste

**Directions:**

1. Mix your onion powder, garlic, powder, sea salt, pepper, cayenne powder, and paprika in a bowl. Stir until well combined.
2. Add your ribs to your mixture, tossing to coat them. Line a baking sheet, arranging your ribs on it.
3. Heat your oven to 325, and then bake for two and a half hours.
4. In a box, mix your paleo friendly BBQ sauce with your raw honey. Stir well, and then add in your sriracha sauce, stirring again.

5. Take your ribs out of the oven, and then baste them with your BBQ sauce mixture. Preheat your grill over medium-high heat, cooking for seven minutes per side.
6. Sprinkle with cilantro, parsley and chives before serving warm.

**Nutrition Facts:**

**Calories:** 120

**Fat:** 6.4 Grams

**Protein:** 6.2 Grams

## Toasted Mandarin Salad

Mandarin oranges are a favorite sweet fruit for many on a paleo diet, and you can include them in a salad too.

**Serves:** 1

**Time:** 5 Minutes

**Ingredients:**

- 2 Cups Spring Greens, Fresh
- ¼ Cup Red Onions, Sliced Thin
- 1 Cup Mandarin Oranges, Drained
- Sea Salt & Black Pepper to Taste

**Directions:**

1. Start by combining your red onion and spring greens, mixing well.
2. Transfer to a salad bowl, topping with your mandarin slices.
3. Drizzle with paleo dressing if desired. Season with sea salt and black pepper before serving.

**Nutrition Facts:**

**Calories:** 120

**Fat:** 2 Grams

**Protein:** 3 Grams

# Mushroom Bisque

**Serves:** 6

**Time:** 1 ½ Hours

**Ingredients:**

- 1 Tablespoon Coconut Oil
- 2 lbs. Mushrooms, Sliced
- 1 Medium Onion, Chopped
- 1 Teaspoon Garlic, Minced
- 5 Cups Vegetable Stock, Low Sodium
- ½ Cup Coconut Milk, Unsweetened
- Sea Salt & Black Pepper to Taste
- 3 Tablespoons Almond Flour

**Directions:**

1. Start by heating your coconut oil over medium-high heat in a heavy stockpot. Add in your garlic once your oil is hot, cooking for one minute. Make sure to stir well so that your garlic doesn't burn.
2. Stir in your mushrooms and onion once your garlic has become fragrant. Cook until your onions are soft and translucent. This should take about six to eight minutes.
3. Whisk in your vegetable stock, brining the mixture to a low simmer.
4. Simmer for an hour, and then get out a small bowl. Whisk your almond flour and coconut milk in the bowl until it's well combined.
5. Whisk your coconut milk mixture into the soup, and then allow it to simmer for five more minutes to thicken slightly. Season with salt and pepper again before serving.

**Nutrition Facts:**

**Calories:** 160

**Fat:** 10 Grams

**Protein:** 5 Grams

# Roasted Rosemary Chicken

Rosemary is a great herb to go with chicken, and it's one of those paleo seasonings that is easy to grow in your own home.

**Serves:** 4

**Time:** 1 Hour

**Ingredients:**

- 2 Carrots, Chopped
- 2 Sweet Potatoes, Chopped
- 1 Onion, Quartered
- 2 lbs. Chicken Thighs, Boneless & Skinless
- 1 Tablespoon Coconut Oil
- 1 Teaspoon Garlic, Minced
- 1 Zucchini, Chopped
- 1 Cup Cauliflower Florets
- ¼ Cup Vegetable Stock
- 2 Tablespoon Dried Rosemary
- 1 Teaspoon Dried Basil
- Sea Salt & Black Pepper to Taste

**Directions:**

1. Start by heating your oven to 400, and then place a large skillet over medium-high heat with your oil and garlic inside.
2. Season your chicken with your sea salt and black pepper before adding it to the skillet.
3. Cook for two to three minutes on each side. Your chicken should be lightly browned when you're done.
4. Combine your vegetables in a baking dish, and then add in your browned chicken. You don't want to mix your chicken in. leave it on the top.

5. Whisk your remaining ingredients together before pouring it over the mixture.
6. Bake for forty-five minutes, cooking until your vegetables are tender.
7. Serve warm.

**Nutrition Facts:**

**Calories:** 710

**Fat:** 50 Grams

**Protein:** 37 Grams

# Turkey & Cilantro Burgers

Cilantro goes great with lean ground turkey, and you can serve these burgers on paleo bread or wrapped in lettuce.

**Serves:** 4

**Time:** 20 Minutes

**Ingredients:**

- 1 ¼ lbs. Ground Turkey, Lean
- ¼ Cup Red Onion, Minced
- ¼ Cup Cilantro, Fresh & chopped
- ½ Teaspoon Chili Powder
- 1 Egg, Beaten
- 2 Tablespoons Almond Flour
- Sea Salt & Black Pepper to Taste

**Directions:**

1. Start by pre-heating your broiler to high heat, and then grease a broiler safe pan.
2. Combine all ingredients in a bowl, stirring well.
3. Shape your mixture into four different patties, placing them in your pan.
4. Broil for three to five minutes. It should be cooked all the way through.
5. Allow to cool slightly before serving.


**Nutrition Facts:**

**Calories:** 300

**Fat:** 15 Grams

**Protein:** 34 Grams

# Stuffed Onions

If you're looking to try something new, then try out this simple stuffed onion recipe. It's both vegetarian and paleo friendly.

**Serves:** 3

**Time:** 35 Minutes

**Ingredients:**

- 3 Onions, Large
- 1 Cup Cauliflower Rice
- 1 Tablespoon Tomato Paste
- 1 Teaspoon Allspice
- 2 Teaspoon Cinnamon
- 1 Teaspoon Cumin
- 1 Teaspoon Coriander
- 1 ½ Teaspoons Sea Salt, Fine
- Coconut Sugar for Topping
- ½ Teaspoon Black Pepper
- 3 Tablespoons Parsley, Fresh & Minced
- 2 Tablespoons Apple Cider Vinegar, With the Mother
- 1 Tablespoon Honey, Raw
- 2 Tablespoons Olive Oil

**Directions:**

1. Start by cutting your cauliflower head into florets. You'll then need to lace them into a boiling pot of water, cooking for fifteen minutes.
2. Once tender, drain your florets and pat them with a clean paper towel. Pulse them together in a food processor.
3. Fill a saucepan with water, bringing it to a boil.
4. Cut the tops of your onion, and then make a small cut into each.

5.  Turn the heat to medium-high, and let your saucepan of water boil.

6.  Once it starts to boil, add in your onions, cooking for ten minutes.

7.  Your cauliflower rice should be drained, and then add then place it into a bowl.

8.  Add your cinnamon, allspice, cumin, tomato paste, coriander, sea salt, pepper and cilantro together.

9.  Remove your onions, letting them cool for five minutes.

10.  Separate the layers of your onions, and then put a tablespoon of filing into each. Wrap the onions back up around the filling.

11. Take an oven safe saucepan, and place it over medium-high heat before adding a tablespoon of olive oil.

12. Once it gets hot, place your onions with the seam down, and then let them cook for one to two minutes.

13. Add in your vinegar, sprinkling coconut sugar over the onions.

14. Cover your pan, cooking for twenty minutes. You'll need to rotate the onions during the cooking process, and then serve while still warm.

**Nutrition Facts:**

**Calories:** 149.1

**Fat:** 3.9 Grams

**Protein:** 3.5 Grams

# Crusted Tilapia

Tilapia is a cheap fish that's easy to get, but it still packs a good bit of flavor. Even more so with this coconut crust.

**Serves:** 4

**Time:** 25 Minutes

**Ingredients:**

- 4 Tilapia Fillets, Boneless & 6 Ounces
- ¼ Cup Coconut Flakes, Unsweetened
- 2 Tablespoons Coconut Flour
- Sea Salt & Black Pepper to Taste

**Directions:**

1. Start by heating your oven to 350, and then grease a baking sheet.
2. Season your fish with salt and pepper before placing them on your baking sheet.
3. Spray your fish down with paleo friendly cooking oil.
4. Combine your coconut flour and coconut together, sprinkling it liberally over your fillets.
5. Cook for twelve to fifteen minutes. The fish should flake easily with a fork.
6. Serve hot.

**Nutrition Facts:**

**Calories:** 220

**Fat:** 7 Grams

**Protein:** 35 Grams

## Perfect Bacon Wrapped Scallops

Simplicity is sometimes best, which you'll find is true with this easy bacon wrapped scallop recipe.

**Serves:** 8

**Time:** 30 Minutes

**Ingredients:**

- 1 ½ lbs. Scallops, Fresh, Rinsed & Patted Dry
- 1 lb. Bacon, Thin Sliced & Uncooked
- ¼ Teaspoon Paprika
- ¼ Teaspoon Chili Powder
- ¼ Teaspoon Sea Salt, Fine
- Black Pepper to Taste

**Directions:**

1. Start by preheating your broiler, using high heat.
2. Combine all spices in a bowl before setting them to the side.
3. Wrap each scallop in a bacon slice, and then secure it with a wooden toothpick.
4. Sprinkle the scallops with your spice mixture, arranging them on your pan.
5. Broil for ten to fifteen minutes. Your bacons should be cooked through, and serve warm.

**Nutrition Facts:**

**Calories:** 350

**Fat:** 26 Grams

**Protein:** 25 Grams

## Chicken with Peppers & Cabbage

Cabbage is an easy way to get all of the fiber you need, and it goes great in this chicken recipe.

**Serves:** 4

**Ingredients:**

- 1 ½ lbs.  Chicken Legs, Bone In
- 3 Tablespoons Chicken Stock, Low Sodium
- 2 Bell Peppers, Sliced
- 1 Small Head Cabbage, Chopped
- 2 Tablespoons Olive Oil, Divided
- Parsley, Fresh & Chopped to Garnish
- Sea Salt & Black Pepper to Taste

**Directions:**

1. Start by heating your oven to 375.
2. Season your chicken liberally with sea salt and pepper, and then place them in a prepared glass baking dish.
3. Arrange your peppers and cabbage on top of your chicken.
4. Whisk all remaining ingredients together before drizzling them over your vegetables.
5. Bake for thirty to forty minutes. Your chicken should be cooked all the way through, and serve warm.


**Nutrition Facts:**

**Calories:** 490

**Fat:** 35 Grams

**Protein:** 23 Grams

# Chia Balls

This is an easy paleo snack or dessert that can be stored for up to three days in the fridge.

**Serves:** 8

**Time:** 15 Minutes

**Ingredients:**

- 8 ½ Ounces Dates
- 3 Ounces Chia Seeds
- 2 Ounces Almonds, Raw
- 3 Tablespoons Cacao Powdered

**Directions:**

1. Place your almonds in a food processor, pulsing until well chopped.
2. Add in all of your remaining ingredients except your cocoa powder, pulsing at a low speed for about two minutes.
3. You'll need to add water as needed to get a dough consistency.
4. Roll your dough into balls, and then roll the balls into cocoa powder.
5. Place in the fridge for about ten minutes before serving.


**Nutrition Facts:**

**Calories:** 90.9

**Fat:** 6.1 Grams

**Protein:** 3 Grams

# Paleo Baked Apples

You know that apples are paleo friendly, but you don't always have to eat them on their own. You can turn your apples into a paleo friendly dessert that's sure to delight the entire family.

**Serves:** 4

**Time:** 40 Minutes

**Ingredients:**

- 4 Medium Apples, Cored
- ¼ Cup Golden Raisins
- 3 Tablespoon Maple Syrup, Pure
- 1 Teaspoon Ground Cinnamon
- 1 Cup Apple Juice, Natural

**Directions:**

1. Start by heating your oven to 350.
2. Arrange your apples into a prepared baking dish.
3. Toss your raisins and cinnamon into your apples.
4. Drizzle your maple syrup over them, and then add your apple juice to the dish.
5. Bake for twelve to fifteen minutes. Your apples should be tender, but make sure that they don't burn.
6. Allow to cool for five minutes before serving.

**Nutrition Facts:**

**Calories:** 170

**Fat:** 0 Grams

**Protein:** 1 Gram

# Blueberry & Apple Crisp

A crisp is a great comfort food, and it's meant to be eaten warm. However, you can eat it room temperature, especially if you want to share!

**Serves:** 4

**Time:** 1 Hour 30 Minutes

**Ingredients:**

**Filling:**

- 3 Gala Apples, Peeled, Cored & Sliced into 1/4 Inch Slices
- 1 Tablespoon Butter
- 1 Teaspoon Lemon Juice, Fresh
- 1 Teaspoon Honey, Raw
- ½ Teaspoon Cinnamon
- ½ Cup Blueberries, Fresh
- Pinch Sea Salt, Fine

**Topping:**

- 1 Cup Almond Flour
- 1 Teaspoon Coconut Flour
- ½ Teaspoons Cinnamon
- ¼ Teaspoon Ground Ginger
- 2 Tablespoons Honey, Raw
- ¼ Teaspoon Sea Salt, Fine

**Directions:**

1. Start by turning your oven to 350, and then grease four ramekins that are six ounces eat. Place all of your filling ingredients in a bowl, tossing to combine.

2.  Distribute the filling into your ramekins. Cover your ramekins with foil, and then bake until the fruit starts to become tender, which will be about five minutes.

3.  To make the topping, combine all of your topping ingredients together.

4.  Remove your foil from the ramekins, and then crumble your topping on top.

5.  Return the ramekins to the oven, cooking until browned and the fruit is tender, which should take about ten more minutes.

6.  Allow to cool before serving warm.

**Nutrition Facts:**

**Calories:** 329

**Fat:** 18 Grams

**Protein:** 1 Gram

## Berry Sorbet

When many people start a paleo diet, it can be easy to miss ice cream. Don't fear! You don't need to give up sweet, cold treats entirely. This triple berry sorbet can help you with your ice cream craving.

**Serves:** 4

**Time:** 3 Hours 30 Minutes

**Ingredients:**

- 1 Cup Strawberries, Fresh
- ½ Cup Honey, Raw
- 1 ½ Cups Water
- 3 Tablespoons Lemon Juice, Fresh
- 1 Cup Blueberries, Fresh
- 1 Cup Raspberries, Fresh

**Directions:**

1. Whisk your honey and water together in a saucepan, placing it over medium heat.
2. Cook until the honey starts to melt, stirring until the mixture is smooth.
3. Stir your berries in, bringing the pan to a boil.
4. Reduce the heat, and then simmer your berries until they soften. This should take about five minutes.
5. Take the mixture off of heat before straining it using a sieve.
6. Stir your lemon juice in, covering and chilling it for three hours.
7. Pour your mixture into your ice cream maker, freezing and churning according to your manufacturer instructions.

**Nutrition Facts:**

**Calories:** 65

**Fat:** 1 Gram

**Protein:** 1 Gram

# Chocolate Chip Cookies

This is another recipe that's been turned paleo friendly so that you can enjoy this delicious comfort food.

**Serves:** 12

**Time:** 1 Hour

**Ingredients:**

- 1 Teaspoon Vanilla Extract, Pure
- ½ Cup Honey, Raw
- 2 ½ Cups Almond flour
- 3 Tablespoons Coconut Oil, Melted
- 2 Eggs, Large
- ¼ Teaspoon Baking Soda
- ¼ Teaspoon Sea Salt, Fine
- 1 Cup Chocolate Chips, Dairy Free

**Directions:**

1. Start by turning your oven to 350, and then line a baking sheet.
2. Combine your baking soda, flour, and sea salt in a bowl. Place it to the side.
3. Beat your honey, egg, vanilla extract and coconut oil together.
4. Beat your dry ingredients into your wet ingredients until its smooth.
5. Fold in your chocolate chips, dropping spoonful's of the batter onto your prepared baking sheet.
6. Bake for eight to twelve minutes depending on how chewy you like your chocolate chip cookies. They should be lightly browned.
7. Allow your cookies to cool for five minutes before transferring them to a cooling rack to finish cooling.

**Nutrition Facts:**

**Calories:** 160

**Fat:** 11 Grams

**Protein:** 4 Grams

# Vanilla Cupcakes

If you have a sweet tooth, these vanilla cupcakes will hit the spot. You can serve with a drizzle of honey instead of icing to keep them paleo friendly.

**Serves:** 24

**Time:** 50 Minutes

**Ingredients:**

- ¼ Cup Coconut Flour, Sifted
- 1 ½ Cups Almond Flour
- 2 Teaspoons Vanilla Extract, Pure
- ¼ Teaspoon Sea Salt, Fine
- 1 ½ Teaspoons Baking Powder
- ½ Cup Honey, Raw
- 5 Eggs, Large
- 2 Egg Whites
- 1 Cup Coconut Milk, Unsweetened

**Directions:**

1. Start by heating your oven to 350, and then line two muffin pans with paper liners.
2. Combine your flours, salt, and baking powder together. Mix it and set it to the side.
3. Beat your eggs, egg whites, coconut milk, vanilla extract and honey together in a different bowl. Make sure it's thoroughly combined.
4. Add your dry ingredients into your wet ingredients, beating together until combined.
5. Spoon your batter into your muffin tins.
6. Bake for twenty-five to thirty minutes. A knife should be able to be inserted into the center and come out clean.

7. Allow to cool for ten minutes before placing them on a cooling rack to finish cooling.

**Nutrition Facts:**

**Calories:** 100

**Fat:** 5 Grams

**Protein:** 3 Grams

# Chocolate Mousse

This light and airy dessert will satisfy any chocolate craving, and it's whipped to perfection to make a delightful texture.

**Serves:** 4

**Time:** 1 Hour 20 Minutes

**Ingredients:**

- 2 Cups Coconut Milk, Unsweetened
- 1 Avocado, Pitted & Sliced
- ¼ Cup Honey, Raw
- 1 Teaspoon Vanilla Extract, Pure
- 2 Tablespoons Cocoa Powder, Unsweetened

**Directions:**

1. Start by combining your cocoa powder, vanilla extract, honey and coconut milk in a food processor. Pulse until blended and smooth.
2. Add in your avocado, pulsing again until it forms a light and creamy texture. It should appear whipped.
3. Spoon into cups, and allow it to chill for at least an hour before serving.

**Nutrition Facts:**

**Calories:** 168

**Fat:** 8 Grams

**Protein:** 1 Gram

## Paleo Brownies

Just because you're going paleo, doesn't mean that you have to give up brownies. This paleo friendly brownie recipe will keep your cravings at bay.

**Serves:** 10

**Time:** 45 Minutes

**Ingredients:**

- ½ Cup Cocoa Powder, Unsweetened
- ½ Cup Coconut Flour, Sifted
- 1 Cup Honey, Raw
- 1 Teaspoon Vanilla Extract, Pure
- 6 Eggs, Large
- Pinch Sea Salt, Fine

**Directions:**

1. Start by heating your oven to 350, and then grease a baking dish.
2. Melt your coconut in the microwave if necessary, and then whisk your melted coconut oil with your cocoa powder. Make sure to whisk until the mixture is smooth.
3. In a different bowl, beat your eggs and honey together. Add in your sea salt and vanilla extract, beating until fluffy.
4. Add your coconut oil mixture into your coconut flour, beating it together.
5. Pour your batter into your dish, cooking for thirty to thirty-five minutes. You should be 2able to insert a toothpick into the center and it come out clean.


**Nutrition Facts:**

**Calories:** 220

**Fat:** 10 Grams

**Protein:** 5 Grams

# Cinnamon & Pecan Coffee Cake & Orange Drizzle

This is an easy recipe that's great for dessert, but you can use it for breakfast in a pinch too since it can be made in advance.

**Serves:** 6

**Time:** 1 Hour 30 Minutes

**Ingredients:**

**Cake:**

- 1 Teaspoon Sea Salt, Fine
- 1 Teaspoon Nutmeg
- 2 Cps Coconut Flour
- 1 Tablespoon Cinnamon
- 3 Tablespoons Baking Powder
- 2 Cups Almond Milk, Unsweetened
- 12 Eggs, Beaten Lightly
- 1 Cup Honey, Raw

**Filling:**

- ¼ Cup Pecans, Chopped
- 1 Tablespoon Cinnamon
- 1 ½ Tablespoon Coconut Flour
- 2 Teaspoon Butter
- 1 ½ Tablespoon Honey, Raw
- Pinch Sea Salt

**Drizzle:**

- 2 Teaspoons Orange Juice, Fresh
- 1/3 Cup Honey, Raw
- 2 Teaspoon Orange Zest

**Directions:**

1. Start by turning your oven to 325.
2. Grease a nine by nine inch pan generously with your butter, and set it to the side.
3. Whisk all of your dry cake ingredients together in a bowl.
4. Whisk all of your wet cake ingredients together in a different bowl.
5. Slowly whisk your dry and wet ingredients for your cake mixture together. Keep whisking until all of your lumps are gone.
6. In another bowl, stir all of your filling ingredients together.
7. Spoon half of your cake batter into your pan, and then top with your pecan filling. Top with your remaining cake batter.
8. Bake for about an hour. A toothpick should be able to be inserted into the middle and come back out clean.
9. While your cake is baking, stir all of your drizzle ingredients together.
10. Allow your cake to cool for fifteen minutes.
11. Top with your orange drizzle before serving.

**Nutrition Facts:**

**Calories:** 662

**Fat:** 20 Grams

**Protein:** 21 Grams

## Mocha Pudding

If you're a coffee lover, then you'll love this chilled mocha treat! It also works as a great pick me up since its rich caffeine too.

**Serves:** 4

**Time:** 2 Hours 20 Minutes

**Ingredients:**

**Pudding:**

- 1/3 Cup Arrowroot Flour
- 1/3 Cup Honey, Raw
- Heavy Pinch Sea Salt, Fine
- 2 ¼ Cup Almond Milk, Unsweetened
- 2 Tablespoons Instant Coffee Granules
- 6 Egg Yolks
- 2 Teaspoons Vanilla
- 2 Tablespoons Butter
- 6 Ounces Paleo Dark Chocolate

**Garnish:**

- 1 Ounce Paleo Dark Chocolate, Grated

**Directions:**

1. Take a medium saucepan, and add in your arrowroot flour, sea salt, honey, almond milk, and instant coffee. Whisk well, and then place it over medium heat, bringing the mixture to a boil.
2. In a bowl, whisk your vanilla and egg yolks together before setting the mixture aside.
3. When your almond milk mix comes to a boil, pour it slowly into your egg yolk mixture while whisking.

4. Return the egg yolk and almond milk mix to your pan, placing it over medium heat. Stir constantly, allowing it to thicken and for bubbles to form.
5. Stir in your butter and dark chocolate, whisking as it melts. Make sure that you do not let it burn.
6. Transfer the pudding to a bowl, letting it chill in the fridge for two hours.
7. Garnish with grated paleo dark chocolate before serving.

**Nutrition Facts:**

**Calories:** 513

**Fat:** 29 Grams

**Protein:** 9 Grams

# Almond Custard with Berries

This is a refined but simple dessert, and it's sure to please the crowd! It's a sweet treat that's simply elegant with a delightfully creamy texture.

**Serves:** 4

**Time:** 3 Hours 15 Minutes

**Ingredients:**

- 2 Cups Almond Milk, Unsweetened
- ½ Cup Honey, Raw
- ½ Teaspoon Lemon Zest
- Pinch Sea Salt, Fine
- 6 Egg Yolks
- 2 Teaspoons Vanilla Extract, Pure

**Garnish:**

- 1 Cup Strawberries, Fresh & Sliced
- 1 Cup Raspberries, Fresh
- 1 Cup Blueberries, Fresh

**Directions:**

1. Start by heating your oven to 325, and then get out four ramekins. Six ounce ramekins work best, and then get out a baking dish that can hold all six.
2. In a saucepan, combine your lemon zest, honey, sea salt and almond milk together over medium heat. Bring it to a gentle boil while stirring often.
3. In a bowl, whisk your egg yolks and vanilla together until well combined.
4. Slowly pour your hot almond mixture into your yolk mixture while still whisking.
5. Strain the mixture, and then pour it into your ramekins.

6. Place the ramekins in the over, filling the rest of the dish with water halfway up the ramekins.

7. Bake until they jiggle a bit in the center, which should take about an hour.

8. Cool for twenty minutes, and then cover them with plastic wrap before putting them in the fridge to chill for two hours.

9. Garnish with berries before serving chilled.

**Nutrition Facts:**

**Calories:** 151

**Fat:** 8 Grams

**Protein:** 5 Grams

# Conclusion

Thank you for reading this book. A paleo DIET IS SUCH A GREAT DIET!

It allows for delicious recipes that nourish the body and soul. Foods that are clean, pure, and perfect for staying in shape. Recipes that encourage weight loss, fill you up for hours at a time, and make you feel better and more energetic. These are all positive aspects of a paleo diet. By eating healthy, unprocessed foods, the way they were intended, you will lose weight, feel healthier, and have more energy. It is one of the healthiest ways to eat. Simply following a paleo plan, eating only when you are hungry, and assuring that your foods contain lean meats, healthy fats, and a great variety of vegetables, you will lose weight and feel better. Take control of your life! A paleo diet will lead you to a healthier, happier life.

 Once again, I would like to thank you for downloading this book and having the patience for going through it.

I do hope that you had just as much fun reading and experimenting the meals as much as I enjoyed writing the book.

From now on, all you are going to need to do is properly follow the rules of Paleo and go ahead to experiment with your very own meal plan!

Stay safe, Stay healthy and God Bless!